MW00942461

The Diabetes Slayer's Handbook

Preventing or Reversing Prediabetes and Type 2 Diabetes

ALAN D. RAGUSO

iUniverse, Inc.
Bloomington

The Diabetes Slayer's Handbook
Preventing or Reversing Prediabetes and Type 2 Diabetes

iUniverse books may be ordered through booksellers or by contacting:

iUniverse
1663 Liberty Drive
Bloomington, IN 47403
www.iuniverse.com
1-800-Authors (1-800-288-4677)

ISBN: 978-1-4759-5003-8 (sc)
ISBN: 978-1-4759-5005-2 (e)
ISBN: 978-1-4759-5004-5 (dj)

Library of Congress Control Number: 2012917096

Printed in the United States of America

iUniverse rev. date: 9/26/2012

Disclaimer

This book is not intended as a substitute for professional medical care.

The information in this book is intended to help you make informed decisions about your health.

Only your doctor can diagnose and treat a medical problem. If you think you have a medical problem, you should seek competent medical help from your doctor or a certified diabetes educator.

Dedication

To Roger Rojo

We all miss you, Roger

Contents

Acknowledgments

I would like to thank the following people:

My son, Douglas, for unknowingly inspiring me to reverse my diabetes; my daughter, Katy, for continually encouraging me to write; Stace, my son-in-law, for the book cover illustrations; my doctor, who never quit believing in me; Megan Eaton for the design work on the "Safe House" illustration; Pat Richmond for the assistance with editing; the Certified Diabetes Educators of Walla Walla, Washington; and my wife, Linda, who has been with me every step of the way.

Last but by no means least, I want to thank my fellow prediabetes, type 1– and type 2–diabetes patients and obese and morbidly obese people.

Introduction

A Book Designed by a Diabetes Patient for Diabetes Patients

This is a motivational book. I'm a type 2 R patient. The *R* stands for *reversed*.

Have you been diagnosed with prediabetes or type 2 diabetes? Do you have a family member or friend struggling with the effects of this disease that we are told is "chronic" or lifelong? The common thought is that you will continue to lose ground to this condition. I was in your shoes for ten years, and I understand what you are going through. But now I'm off all medication, and I've been off diabetic medications for two years. My A1C, glucose-monitor readings, fasting-glucose readings, cholesterol, triglycerides, and blood pressure, along with weight changes and muscle development, have been stunning. I've experienced a remarkable turnaround.

If you are tired of being frightened, confused, and frustrated, then please read on.

I grew up knowing that diabetes was prevalent in my family. Also, I battled excess weight all of my life. When my physician started seeing me, I'd already taken some weight off, but I was morbidly obese. After the age of forty, my excess weight became increasingly worse. When I was in my mid-forties, my weight hit 350 pounds.

In January 2001, you wouldn't get a diagnosis of "prediabetic." You were either diabetic or you weren't. When I was forty-eight, I was diagnosed with type 2 diabetes. Since mid-December 2009, I've moved my weight downward from the morbidly obese category, past the two-hundred-pound milestone. I'm now simply overweight and have just about thirty pounds to go to get myself to a healthy weight.

Over time, I watched my diabetes progressively get worse. Eventually, I was taking a load of diabetes medications and developing the early stages of retinopathy (eye damage). I learned that the leading cause of blindness in the United States is diabetes.

Finally, a few years ago, I reached a point when I decided that enough was enough! I had gone on various diets to lose weight, hoping to "control" my diabetes better. I tried an ovo-lacto vegetarian diet, which allowed me to eat eggs and dairy but no meat or fish. In about a year and a half, I only lost three pounds. Four years ago, I went on a strict vegan diet for a year—and lost two pounds. I was sick and miserable. And, if I didn't take handfuls of stomach pills, I suffered from horrible diarrhea. This is not something I was eager to share with anybody, but I had my doctor and pharmacist check into side effects. Neither one could find anything in the chemical make-up of my medications that would cause diarrhea.

In short, I spent years studying nutrition and trying to make sense of why I was so sick—all the while, type 2 diabetes was chipping away at my health daily.

Now, I am compelled to speak out!

Could my story be yours or your loved one's?

You may be asking whether your insulin level really is that bad. There's a good chance that it is not.

Insulin has a job to do. Tissue and muscle cells that are swollen and inflamed may interfere with this job. These cells do not respond to signals from the insulin. Imagine a satellite dish that is full of debris; it won't receive the transmissions from the satellite. You don't need more satellites; you need to realign and clean up the receiver dishes!

Try cleaning up your cells. Cell inflammation can be caused by food allergies. Allergies can also trigger symptoms of IBS (irritable bowel syndrome), which can raise the levels of your glucose and your A1C. The A1C measures how much glucose is stuck to a protein called hemoglobin inside the red blood cells. This means that nutrients aren't absorbed well by your intestines, and you can eat heavily but still, in a sense, "starve"! Stress can also increase your glucose and A1C levels. Fat, tissue, and muscle cells can't work properly if they are swollen and inflamed.

The standard of just maintaining an A1C level of 7 percent or lower will never allow you to get well. A level of 6 percent or lower makes more sense and greatly reduces your risk of complications. Talk with your doctor about setting your A1C target level lower.

If you are reading this book, you want answers to your diabetes questions. If you know what questions to ask, your doctor and diabetes support staff can help you. My approach is designed to help support your doctor, your diabetes educators, and you as you seek those answers.

I feel that withholding medical information that I have learned and that can be potentially life changing for other patients would be ethically and morally wrong.

I believe that, to become healthier, you need to have an understanding of the basics of prediabetes, type 2 diabetes, excess weight, sugar, and metabolism. A common thread connects the weight problem with type 2 diabetes. You can cut that thread and then watch the results.

I hope to give you from my perspective, as a patient who fought and beat both type 2 diabetes and morbid obesity, an understanding of these issues.

"Convergence" is the combination of successful recurring principles. Certain concepts regarding carbohydrates, sugars, and exercise are keys to good health.

Have you ever taken a math class where the basic concepts and definitions were not carefully explained to you? Did you find the course frustrating and confusing? Did you finish the class saying to yourself, *I'm not going through that again*? Don't let that happen to you regarding your health.

If you don't gain an understanding of why your body is malfunctioning, then you will never have a very good chance of making yourself healthy.

In the pages that follow, I will explain these concepts:

Metabolism: Metabolism is the conversion of food into living material and into energy and how your body burns calories.

Diabetes: I will give you a simple definition and some very important things you need to understand in order to reverse your diabetes. Diabetes is a condition where your body has trouble using glucose (blood sugar).

Sugar and carbohydrates: Are they villains? Or is there something about them that can make them safe to consume for diabetics? What's the relationship of sugar to prediabetes, type 2 diabetes, and excess weight?

This book offers a game plan for attacking prediabetes, type 2 diabetes, and excess weight; knowing the components inside and out can lead you to your new lifestyle.

The Terrorist

How can you fight something you don't understand? Defending yourself from something you can't see indeed seems impossible. We can discuss your options.

I had been referred to an ophthalmologist due to my worsening eye condition. As I drove home, I was angry and scared. *How did this happen?* I wondered. What was I really going to do about it?

I'd been fighting diabetes for about nine years, and my condition just kept getting worse. I'd developed the disease early in 2001, the year of 9/11. It was the year of the terrorist. Then it hit me: *Diabetes is a terrorist.* It will maim and kill as many people as possible. It had killed several of my friends and family. I then realized *you don't negotiate with a terrorist!* You take out the terrorist before it takes you out. I decided to declare total war on the terrorist!

I set out on a plan to lose weight and try to control my diabetes. Little did I know that I would stumble onto some incredibly simple solutions, ways to win the war I was fighting against raging diabetes, morbid obesity, high blood pressure, high cholesterol, high triglyceride levels, joint and tissue pain, diarrhea, and fatigue.

The Assault on Diabetes

How do you fight a condition like prediabetes or type 2 diabetes?

It takes some time and patience, but the payoff is well worth it. You have to "pay for the bus ride," but, man—what a ride!

I came off of all my diabetes medications in ten months, after being on them for almost ten years.

The keys to your victory over prediabetes, type 2 diabetes, and excess weight are to have

- the means;
- the will; and
- the knowledge.

In World War II, two famous tank commanders faced off against each other. Each was determined to annihilate the other in battle. One was General Erwin Rommel of Germany; the other was General George C. Patton of the United States.

Eventually, General Patton defeated Rommel in battle. Why? I feel that there were three key elements of General Patton's success: First, he had the *means*. The third army was at his disposal. By far, it was the top-of-the-line fighting group. Second, he had the *will*. He didn't get "blood and guts Patton" fame by being weak or giving up.

Finally, he had that final element that is so necessary in defeating a strong enemy. That element is *knowledge*. He studied Rommel's writings and learned how the German general thought. Patton found Rommel's weak points and exploited them.

Find your enemy's weak point, exploit that weak point, and hit the enemy from all sides! Once you know how to defeat diabetes, you can proceed to do so.

Learn all you can about your diabetes condition. Ask your doctor about getting plugged into diabetes education, support groups, workshops, and other specialized diabetes exercise and education programs. Only about 26 percent of prediabetes and type 2–diabetes patients attend diabetes-education programs. Train yourself for war. Whether you realize it or not, you *are* at war. Attend as many educational training sessions as you can. You—and only you—have to decide how well you want to be!

Victimized

Do you feel intimidated and embarrassed about having prediabetes or type 2 diabetes? I felt victimized by this cowardly disease. It attacks soft targets such as nerves, blood vessels, eyes, feet, and kidneys. The majority of amputations in the United States are diabetes related.

One place to start is by looking at your diet. Your body is designed to be a racecar. Your muscles are your high-powered racing engine. What are you going to put in the fuel tank—high-octane racing fuel or stove oil? The stove oil will plug up your fuel lines and eventually seize up the engine. Processed carbohydrates and sugars are like stove oil. Naturally dense carbohydrates and natural sugars such as fructose that is found in fresh fruits are like high-octane fuel for your body.

Once you understand what's going on with your body and the simple things you can do to help make yourself well again, you can set out to do just that: Get well again. You will be able to successfully engage in nutritional and exercise warfare against diabetes and obesity!

So what if you don't produce much insulin? You won't need much insulin if you make minor adjustments in your lifestyle. So what if you have insulin resistance? You can fix that problem too!

My system promotes a healthy lifestyle "transition." I spent ten years taking prescription drugs to force my pancreas to squeeze out extra insulin. My pancreas has been on vacation for two years now! If only I'd figured out years ago what to do, I could have stopped taxing my pancreas with all those medications.

Payback

Fellow patients have often asked me why I'm so passionate about destroying diabetes. It's simple. Diabetes has killed some of my friends and family. I was not able to help them, and I felt sick and helpless. My passion is a desire for payback! I want other diabetes patients to get well and to join in the war against diabetes. We have a responsibility to help ourselves and then move on to help others.

What often gives me the strength to continue on with my war on diabetes is the enthusiasm I see in other patients when they understand what their problem is and learn solutions for their problems.

I realize that we are all different. No two patients have the same health conditions. But deep down, we all want to be healthy and happy.

Diabetes is one of the most confusing and misunderstood diseases in existence. But being diagnosed with prediabetes or type 2 diabetes is not a death sentence unless you ignore it or aren't diagnosed with it until you're seriously ill and have serious medical complications.

I want to see the day that diabetes is eradicated from the face of the earth.

Change Your Health Destiny

I spent eight years believing that my type 2 diabetes was a result of heredity, that my weight condition was hopeless, and that, at best, I could only hope to barely contain diabetes. Slowly this disease would "chip away at me" until eventually I would face serious medical complications.

Faced with the early stages of retinopathy, I had to make a decision. I could roll over and submit to the concept that I couldn't defeat diabetes—or I could do something dramatic to fight and reverse this disease. I chose to fight! You can do the same. Many of you can do things to take back your health and be in command again of your life.

At age sixty, I'm in better health in some respects than I was at age thirty. I've been off all diabetes medication for two years now. For that matter, I'm actually off of *all* medications.

For economic reasons alone, this bear's shouting out! I am no longer standing, hat in hand, waiting in line for my drugs, and I'm eating everyday foods! The cost savings are fantastic.

Your Doctor

Really talk to your doctor. Ask your doctor what it will take for you to get well. Don't just discuss "controlling" diabetes. Talk about *reversing* it. An A1C level that is just under 7.0 may not get you well, and maintaining that level could put you at risk for diabetes complications. Ask your doctor about getting your A1C below 6.0 percent. Of course, you always should consult your physician before starting any diet or exercise program.

Do not ever change or stop taking any of your medications without your doctor's permission. I recommend following your doctor's instructions, as I do.

Diabetes Education Is the Key

Talk frequently with your doctor, certified diabetes educators (CDEs), and dieticians. CDEs have extensive medical training and medical experience.

CDEs must have many hours of training and extensive medical knowledge to be certified to work with prediabetes, type 1–, and type 2–diabetes patients. I salute the CDEs; they're in the trenches in the war against diabetes.

Work with your doctor and CDEs. Take a team approach for success in beating diabetes. Tell your doctor what *you* want.

Only about a quarter of prediabetes and type 2 diabetes patients attend even one education class.

This is unfortunate and leads to misconceptions. I've heard the comment from diabetics that "there isn't anything I can eat." This is far from the truth; there is an incredible range of foods you can eat. Education classes can help you find out what those foods are.

Although the general guideline used is aiming for an A1C of less than 7.0 percent, I suggest that you ask your doctor about getting your A1C under 6.0 percent. Push to get yourself under prediabetic levels—that means 5.7 percent or lower.

A1C to eAG Conversion Chart

Use this A1C to eAG conversion chart as a reference. You can't know where you're going if you don't know where you are.

This table shows the relationship between A1C and eAG (estimated average glucose).

A1C percent	eAG mg/dl
5	97
5.5	111
6	126
6.5	140
7	154
7.5	169
8	183
8.5	197
9	212
9.5	226
10	240
10.5	255
11	269

Three points on your glucose monitor equals a tenth of a percentage point on your A1C level. If my monitor were to register 111, I would know that the A1C equivalent is 5.5.

If, for example, you had two separate glucose readings of 120 and 140, you would add those together and divide by 2. You would get an average of 130, which is about a 6.2 A1C equivalent.

The Sinking Ship

The year 2012 marked the one hundredth anniversary of the sinking of the *Titanic*. We remember the horrific tragedy and that many lives were lost. We forget that a sizable number of passengers survived.

Let me ask you a question. That evening, if you had sensed that something was seriously wrong, would you have sat down in the lower section of the ship arranging silverware and waiting for the midnight buffet? Would you instead have opted to leave the warmth of the ship interior and wind your way up numerous stairs out into the cold air to find a life jacket, put it on, and wait for the possibility that a lifeboat would be unlashed and lowered so that you might be lucky enough to get into it? Remember, it was very cold out. You'd have been cold and uncomfortable—but you might have felt the need to do this to survive.

Imagine that you did this. Other people would still be down inside the warm ship. Standing there by yourself, would you have wondered whether you had made the right decision? What if, just then, you heard the scraping of an iceberg against the side of the ship? Somehow, you'd know you were right.

Taking action before it is too late may just save your life.

The Metabolic Syndrome

Prediabetes, type 2 diabetes, excess weight, high blood pressure, high LDL (bad cholesterol levels), low HDL (good cholesterol levels), and high triglyceride levels—together, these create the "metabolic syndrome."

Basically, it means that you're getting painted into a corner with multiple risks to your health.

I have found that the majority of prediabetes and type 2–diabetes patients who are referred to diabetes counseling, diabetes workshops, diabetes support-group meetings, and prediabetes combined exercise and education programs have been newly diagnosed with their condition, have control problems, or have risk factors, a term that generally refers to the metabolic syndrome.

Originally, I sought to lose weight and assumed that I would have to lose a certain amount of weight to get my diabetes under control. What I didn't realize was that the system that I developed attacked the metabolic syndrome—battling most of our major health concerns—like a vicious junkyard dog!

Diabesity

Diabesity is a term used by diabetes experts to refer to the combination of diabetes and obesity. It acknowledges the connection between obesity or morbid obesity and diabetes.

Controlling the absorption of refined sugars and carbohydrates is the key to controlling both diabetes and excess weight.

I hate the term *obesity*. The word makes me feel like something that was scraped off the bottom of somebody's shoe. Instead of calling excess weight *obesity*, we should use a numbered rating scale, as we do with hurricanes.

The principle is simple: excess sugar absorbed into the bloodstream leads to weight gain, and a decrease in sugar leads to weight loss.

Some people can be overweight and not have diabetes, while others may have diabetes and not be substantially overweight.

I realized that the same thing that is responsible for excess weight—excess absorbed sugar in the bloodstream—is also responsible for prediabetes and type 2 diabetes. That sugar has to be burned up as fuel in the muscles or stored as energy in the fat cells. Otherwise, it remains floating in your bloodstream, causing problems for your blood vessels.

I fought excess weight all of my life. In our society, an unspoken phrase that often comes to mind when we see seriously overweight people is "they're fat and lazy."

But when I see a morbidly obese person, the first thing that hits me is a wave of sadness. The second thing that occurs is that I think, "That person's cell system is poisoned." Finally, I have the realization that the problem can be fixed.

A Word about Weight

Not all prediabetics and type 2 diabetics are significantly overweight, and not all overweight, obese, and morbidly obese individuals are prediabetics or have type 2 diabetes. We need to remember that we are all different, and we all have different combinations and degrees of medical conditions.

Regardless of what you're fighting (excess weight, prediabetes, or type 2 diabetes) you will find the *sugar connection*. Sugar absorbed into your bloodstream must be burned for energy; if it remains in your bloodstream, it will eventually cause health problems or be carried to your fat cells to be stored as—you guessed it—more fat.

Don't try to lose weight to satisfy your ego. Don't try to lose weight for a special event, such as a high school reunion. Lose weight to improve your health.

Initially, you may lose weight rapidly, but eventually the weight loss will slow down. You may even hit a plateau where your weight doesn't go down for some time. You might also experience a "weight rebound"—which means that you might gain some weight back after losing a lot of weight. Relax and be patient. You eventually will start losing weight again.

You need to lose your weight slowly. The weight loss will be more permanent if it's done slowly. I'd rather take five years to lose all my excess weight than lose it quickly, only for it to come back and stay with me forever. Ask yourself where you want to be one year, two years, and five years from now. Adopt a long-term weight-loss plan. And *don't give up! You will win!*

You need to burn an extra 3,500 calories to lose one pound of weight. Conversely, weight gain occurs when you consume too many calories. *Just a net change of 100 calories per day can add up to ten pounds in a year.*

Many obese individuals can easily reduce their daily calorie intake by 1,000 calories without feeling deprived!

There's an arsenal of delicious foods available—inexpensive, everyday items that you can easily find right in your grocery store.

Sleep—or the Lack of It

Studies indicate that most people should have eight and a half hours of sleep every night for good health. It's very hard to get that much sleep every night and still balance work, family, hobbies, errands, and, last but not least, exercise. I try for seven and a half hours of sleep per night. It's not perfect, but we are not in a perfect world.

Without proper sleep, our minds can't reorganize and our bodies can't heal properly.

Lack of sleep can adversely affect your blood-glucose levels as well. When you are tossing and turning in bed, getting up and down through the night, or just plain staying up too late, you pay a price when it comes to diabetes and excess weight.

Our body puts out hormones early in the morning to activate us, but those hormones can interfere with our processing of insulin.

Many prediabetics and type 2 diabetics have their greatest glucose control problems when they wake up in the morning.

I find that if I reduce the amount of carbohydrates, especially refined carbohydrates, that I consume after dinner, my early morning glucose tends to be lower, requiring less exercise in the morning to reduce any slight elevations in my glucose. While I no longer need to use glucose test strips, I do occasionally take random test samples so that I can relate to other patients.

Glucose Spikes and Dawn Phenomenon: Tips to Avoid Them

It is very important to regulate your post-meal glucose levels after dinner at night. High glucose levels at night can continue until you get up the next morning. That's a lot of hours of high glucose levels, and it can ruin your A1C level readings!

Read your food labels! You can't control the amount of sugar hitting your bloodstream if you don't have any idea how many grams of refined carbohydrates and sugars you're consuming. If you load up on foods that convert to blood sugar quickly, of course you will get a glucose spike.

One of the biggest mistakes that many people make is consuming too much food in the evening—in particular, consuming too much of the *wrong* foods late in the evening. Doing so sets the stage for an ugly glucose reading in the morning.

You can use chlorophyll to get your muscle and tissue cells to be less insulin-resistant. Increasing your metabolism will burn more sugar. And, if you time and control your consumption of processed carbohydrates and sugars, you will see surprising and fast changes occur in your glucose readings. This might sound like "playing tricks" on your body. So what if it is? All's fair in war. Remember that you are at war with diabetes, and you want to come out the winner, not the loser.

You've Got to Pay for the Bus Ride

If you insist on believing that you have a chronic (lifelong) disease and that your condition will only get worse, then you probably will get sicker over time.

You have to "believe to achieve"! I encourage you to try visualization.

Visualization allows you to see how your body works and aids your continuing success in defeating prediabetes or type 2 diabetes, or winning your battle with excess weight. You will be able to see things in a new light.

You have to believe that you will get healthier over time. Don't just look at days and weeks; think in terms of months and years. Where do you want to be five years from now? Do you want to be able to move about freely and not be debilitated? The journey to better health is in your hands.

You have to be willing to make the effort to get healthy. It *is* up to you. Before you get on the bus, *you've got to pay for the ride.*

Poker

Imagine that you've been at a casino table for several hours playing poker, a game where you don't really know the rules. The card dealer is sharp and fast. You keep losing—one big hand after another. Oh, sure, once in a while you win a small pot, but then you go back to losing big hands again. The dealer smiles.

Suddenly, the casino manager bursts through the door, accompanied by several security guards. The card dealer is whisked away, and the casino manager explains to you that you've been taken advantage of. The dealer was using a marked deck of cards. Add to that the fact that you didn't know how to play poker in the first place, and you didn't stand a chance.

The casino manager wants to make it up to you. All of your losses will be returned to you—plus, you'll be given an additional 20 percent if you just stay in the game. If you lose that extra 20 percent, you will be back to your original break-even amount, and you can simply go home and have not lost any money. The manager explains the rules of poker. A new dealer starts to deal the cards. (A fresh, clean deck has been opened, and a reputable dealer is now dealing the cards.) You start winning. First you draw two of a kind. Then, the next hand, you win the pot with a straight. Again, you win with a flush. You really start to like this game. Your chips are piling up. You are a winner!

The same goes for diabetes and your health. You just have to know the game and have a fair chance to win.

The Food Groups

Carbohydrates—Carbohydrates consist of sugar (unrefined and refined), starches, other fibers, and sugar alcohols.

You will often hear of the "starchy" foods. These foods are quick to break down into sugars after they are eaten, especially if they are heavily cooked and/or processed. They include breads, cereals, and grains; starchy vegetables, such as potatoes; crackers, chips, and snack foods; and legumes, such as beans, peas, and lentils.

I am not afraid to consume legumes when they are in their natural, "dense" carbohydrate form. They will turn to sugar much more slowly than highly processed foods. Avoid packaged products with added flavoring, cheeses, and sauces. That's where you can get into trouble with your glucose control.

I group carbohydrates into two groups: "spikers" (a "spike" is a glucose-reading increase greater than 50) that rapidly turn into blood sugar, and "stabilizers," which are slow to be absorbed into the bloodstream.

Fruits—In their natural, raw form, quick-frozen, or canned (without sugar), fruits will improve your health and help reverse your diabetes.

I avoid canned fruits, though, even if they are in natural fruit juices instead of added syrup. They turn to sugar faster than fresh or frozen fruit because they have been precooked, which eliminates some of the digestive process.

Diabetics should also avoid fruit juice, which is high in sugar and low in fiber. Instead, try "diet" fruit juices, which are high in flavor and very low in carbohydrates and calories. There are fruit beverages out there that are extremely low in carbohydrates and calories; they won't spike your glucose.

Milk—While milk has a lot of nutrients, it is also high in carbohydrates and calories. Compare the food labels of milk and unsweetened almond beverages. You will be shocked.

Sweets, desserts, and other carbohydrates—Travel through this one like you are walking through a minefield. *Very carefully!*

Non-starchy vegetables—These should be at the top of your list. Green leafy vegetables have virtually no carbohydrates, and they are loaded with chlorophyll. They also have substantial amounts of fiber, which helps slow the absorption of sugar and gives you a feeling of fullness. And, yes, even the lowly iceberg lettuce plays a part in the battle plan to defeat diabetes.

Proteins—Meat, fish, and nuts give you the building blocks to repair tissue. Also, they slow the absorption of sugar into your bloodstream.

Fats—Eat plenty of good fats, in particular omega-3 fats, but avoid the unhealthy omega-6 fats.

Alcohol—Limit your intake of alcohol; it is high in carbohydrates.

Some experts recommend that you consume between 120 and 160 grams of carbohydrates per day. I'm fine with that recommendation, but I suggest limiting the daily intake of processed carbohydrates to 30 grams *per day*. The rest of your carbohydrates should be natural, dense carbohydrates that are slow to break down into sugar. When reading a food label, look for

- the amount of net digestible carbohydrates;

- the amount of calorie content in the food serving; and

- the saturated (bad) fat content.

Once again, I want to emphasize that the ideal diet, which I will introduce in the next chapter, is not a low-carbohydrate diet. The type and quantity of *certain types* of carbohydrates that diabetics consume makes the difference. Also, a healthful diet includes plenty of healthy fats and protein, which helps keep the body balanced.

My recommendations are not a sprint; you will not achieve miraculous results in ninety days. Yes, you will see some results immediately, but remember, this is a marathon that you will be running for the rest of your life. This is a lifestyle *transition*. I encourage you to gradually make changes that you can stay with for the rest of your life.

The MAID:
Mediterranean Anti-inflammation Diet

The MAID is based on eating a combination of healthful complex carbohydrates (natural and dense), natural sugars, healthful fats (omega-3 fatty acids), and lean protein.

Diabetes and obesity cannot survive in the "Safe House" (see diagram). You can venture out of the Safe House occasionally. Diabetes and obesity will be out there waiting for you—but they won't be able to attack you when you're back in the Safe House. If they follow you in there, they will wither and die.

Eat when you are hungry! Don't eat what you like; like what you eat. It takes three weeks to develop a habit. Check with your doctor, diabetes educator, or dietician regarding this program before starting it.

The MAID is both a Mediterranean diet and an anti-inflammation diet. Timing is everything. The MAID uses the concept of glycemic load, which goes beyond the glycemic index and takes into account the volume of the food along with its glycemic index (a measure of how quickly foods convert to sugar in your bloodstream).

You *don't* need complicated math to follow this plan! Simply count from one to thirty processed carbohydrates between noon and 8:00 p.m. If you want to vary the time period somewhat, go ahead. Just watch your glucose readings for spikes (higher-than-normal glucose increases).

Any carbohydrates and sugars that you consume need to be absorbed, burned as fuel, or stored as fat—or they will be left in your bloodstream, where large amounts can cause havoc.

Chlorophyll comes from plants, just as protein comes from animals and nuts. We need both for good health. When you think of chlorophyll, think green. You want to "eat green."

Our bodies build up toxins from our environment and from the foods we eat. Toxins and yeasts build up in our tissue cells, making them swollen and inflamed. The cells can become insulin-resistant. Chlorophyll helps to clean out those toxins and yeasts from our cells.

Capsaicin, an element in spicy or "hot" foods, tends to rev up our metabolism. Peppers contain capsaicin, which has various health benefits for people with prediabetes and type 2 diabetes. Capsaicin revs up the brown fat cells in our body; these cells regulate the burning of energy in our bodies. It seems that capsaicin causes white fat cells, which normally don't metabolize, to become hybrid cells with mitochondria that, in essence, metabolize. Fat is released from the cells, and our body's enzymes remove them from our body. Neat trick, I'd say. Capsaicin prevents the release of insulin for about thirty minutes after consumption.

The MAID diet is not a low-carbohydrate, low-fat, or high-protein diet. Everything is balanced. The MAID is healthful for the whole family.

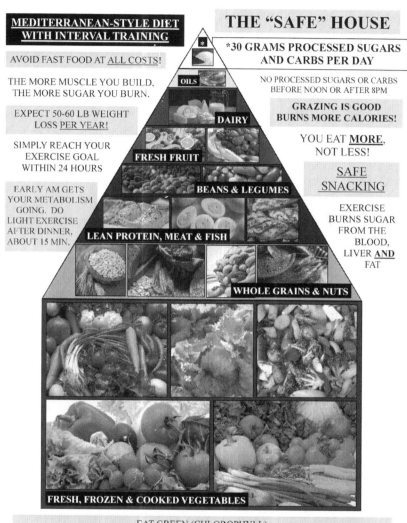

MEDITERRANEAN-STYLE DIET WITH INTERVAL TRAINING

AVOID FAST FOOD AT ALL COSTS!

THE MORE MUSCLE YOU BUILD, THE MORE SUGAR YOU BURN.

EXPECT 50-60 LB WEIGHT LOSS PER YEAR!

SIMPLY REACH YOUR EXERCISE GOAL WITHIN 24 HOURS

EARLY AM GETS YOUR METABOLISM GOING. DO LIGHT EXERCISE AFTER DINNER, ABOUT 15 MIN.

THE "SAFE" HOUSE

*30 GRAMS PROCESSED SUGARS AND CARBS PER DAY

NO PROCESSED SUGARS OR CARBS BEFORE NOON OR AFTER 8PM

GRAZING IS GOOD BURNS MORE CALORIES!

YOU EAT **MORE**, NOT LESS!

SAFE SNACKING

EXERCISE BURNS SUGAR FROM THE BLOOD, LIVER **AND** FAT

OILS

DAIRY

FRESH FRUIT

BEANS & LEGUMES

LEAN PROTEIN, MEAT & FISH

WHOLE GRAINS & NUTS

FRESH, FROZEN & COOKED VEGETABLES

EAT GREEN (CHLOROPHYLL)

CAPCAICIN (METABOLIZE THE BROWN FAT CELLS **AND** THE WHITE FAT CELLS)

Cornerstones of the Mediterranean Anti-inflammation Diet

The Safe House illustrates a diet that combines a Mediterranean-style diet with an anti-inflammation diet. The two diets are blended together and combined with simple kinds of exercise to yield stunning results in combating prediabetes, type 2 diabetes, and excess weight or obesity.

There are some key elements to the Safe House (see illustration). You will notice that the base or foundation of the house is composed of vegetables. How many processed carbohydrates are found in fresh, raw, or cooked vegetables? Virtually none. How many processed carbohydrates will you find in plain, quick-frozen vegetables? Again, you will find virtually none. The chlorophyll in vegetables helps to clean out your tissue and muscle cells of chemical toxins and yeasts. In addition, phytochemicals found in fruits and vegetables have a magic benefit that goes beyond the regular health benefits and diabetes-fighting benefits we think of when we eat vegetables. The powerful phytochemicals are essential elements in cancer prevention. "Eating your fruits and vegetables" never had so much importance as it does now. Weight reversal or maintenance, diabetes reversal, reducing high blood pressure, improving levels of cholesterol and triglycerides, reducing joint and tissue pain, fighting heart attacks and strokes, and, last but not least, helping fight cancer—all from eating vegetables. How much fiber do you think you'll find in vegetables? Lots of it! Fiber helps clean out your digestive system, and it slows or blocks the absorption of processed carbohydrates and processed sugars. In addition, vegetables help keep you feeling full and satisfied. *I do not count the calories of the vegetables I eat. Sugar alcohols that are derived from vegetables are slowly absorbed into the bloodstream.*

Whole grains and nuts are positioned next in the Safe House. They are full of nutrients, fiber, protein, vitamins, minerals, and dense, natural carbohydrates—unless they have been altered by processing for fast-food preparation. Also, you will find the good fats containing omega-3 fatty acids in nuts. These will help you increase your "good" cholesterol (HDL) while reducing your "bad" cholesterol (LDL). They will help slow the absorption of processed carbohydrates and sugars. Corn is high in calories and carbohydrates, and I recommend avoiding it. *I count the calories in grains and nuts.*

An important note: You need to track the grams of processed carbohydrates and processed sugars that you consume. Remember to confine consumption of these to mid- and late daytime. You also need to track your calorie intake. The two are *connected!*

Set up a comprehensive attack plan with your doctor, registered dietician, or certified diabetes educator. The more CDEs you are working with, the better; some dieticians are CDEs.

Lean protein, primarily meat and fish, is at the next level of the Safe House. Protein helps your body's cells repair themselves. Also, protein will help reduce the absorption of processed carbohydrates and sugars into your bloodstream.

My suggestion is to have at least two or three servings of fish per week. Cold-water fish, such as salmon and tuna, are rich in omega-3 fatty acids (the good guys). Eggs and cheese are also part of the protein category. Consuming six eggs per week can help ward off potential eye damage. White cheeses, such as part-skim, low-fat mozzarella cheese, are the healthiest for you. *I count these calories.*

Nuts are also a good source of protein. Walnuts, almonds, and hazelnuts are full of omega-3 fatty acids as well as monounsaturated and polyunsaturated fats. Soy is a good source of protein that most people can tolerate. If you're not allergic to it, certainly incorporate it into your daily diet intake.

Beans and legumes come in next. They are sometimes referred to as "starchy" foods. They are rich in vitamins, minerals, and nutrients, along with fiber. They make a good substitute for meats and heavy starch items, such as potatoes, corn, and hominy.

I count these calories.

The fresh fruit category goes hand in hand with vegetables. Fruits are full of vitamins, minerals, nutrients, phytochemicals, and fiber. These foods contain fructose, or fruit sugar, which is slowly absorbed into the bloodstream. Citrus juices, along with natural unseasoned vinegars, neutralize sugars. Dried fruits are convenient and full of nutrients, but they are also high in sugar. Eat them in small quantities; think of ten raisins as ten grapes.

I count these calories.

Dairy products and yogurt have a lot of nutritional value as well as being a protein source. Low-fat and nonfat yogurt or milk is a good source for many vitamins and minerals. However, you have to consider the sugar. I use an unsweetened almond beverage drink, which is full of vitamins, nutrients, and antioxidants, instead of milk. It has about one-third the calories of milk and has about one net gram of carbohydrate content—as compared with milk's thirteen grams of carbohydrates. You can find unsweetened almond beverages that are free of dairy, soy, lactose, cholesterol, peanuts, casein, gluten, eggs, saturated fat, and MSG. An almond beverage has about 50 percent more calcium than milk and is rich in vitamins D and E. It has a low glycemic index and is vegan.

I count these calories.

Definitely count calories from oils, including monounsaturated and polyunsaturated, such as olive, canola, walnut, and almond oils.

Omega-3 fatty acids found in fish oil, olive oil, canola oil, and walnuts and almonds help fight the effects of cortisol, which increases our levels of unhealthy abdominal fat.

My most important recommendation is to limit yourself to thirty grams of processed carbohydrates and sugars per day. And—this is really important—consume those thirty grams when you are the most active. This is, for most people, between noon and 8:00 p.m. During these hours, you have the best ability to burn up carbohydrates and sugars.

This diet plan utilizes the Harvard Medical School's "Glycemic Load" concept. It takes into account the quality and quantity of the carbohydrates you consume.

Let's discuss spikers and stabilizers with regard to carbohydrates. As stated above, spikers are carbohydrates that rapidly raise your blood-glucose levels. A spike is a glucose increase of 50 or more points on your glucose monitor. Stabilizers are carbohydrates that slowly raise glucose levels.

Do you think that a carb is a carb is a carb? That is not exactly true. You can time and control the amount of carbohydrates and sugars that are absorbed into your bloodstream.

The Economics of the MAID

Following the MAID plan will save you money. First, you can reduce food costs by dining out less often at restaurants and fast-food outlets. As you decrease or eliminate medications, you will also save money. Cost savings may also result if you need fewer dental and eye exams and lab tests as your health improves. Besides saving money, think of the time you will save by having fewer such procedures and needing to spend less time in the pharmacy line.

On top of all of that, your peace of mind will be greatly enhanced and you may find that you take fewer sick days from work.

If that's not enough motivation, following the MAID plan might increase your energy, enabling you to accomplish many more tasks and be much more effective throughout the course of a day.

You might just feel that you have turned back your age clock by years, possibly decades.

Counting Processed Carbohydrates and Processed Sugars

Do you think that a carb is a carb is a carb? Not so fast!

The three basic building blocks of food are proteins, fats, and carbohydrates. For now, let's talk about carbohydrates or "carbs." You will find that carbohydrates can be divided up into sugars, fiber, and sugar alcohols, which are refined sugars from vegetation that are slowly absorbed into the bloodstream. When calculating net carbohydrates, you'll want to subtract fiber and sugar alcohol from the total number of grams of carbohydrates that you have consumed.

A myth exists that says that all carbohydrates are the same. That's not exactly the case. Some carbohydrates and certain sugars will be absorbed into your bloodstream much faster than others. Once you understand this concept, you will be able to turn the tide against diabetes.

The term "glycemic load" refers to how quickly a given volume of carbohydrates will convert to sugar in the bloodstream. When I talk about sugar absorption, I am talking about sugar that goes into the bloodstream. This sugar is fine as long as it's burned up for fuel by the body's muscles or tissues. However, any sugar that is not burned up either will be stored in your fat cells, making you fatter, or it will simply remain floating around in your bloodstream, creating havoc with your health.

Get the monkey off your back! This refers to carbohydrate and sugar addiction. Instead of snacking on starchy or sugary foods, choose natural and dense carbohydrates and natural sugars, such as the fructose found in fresh fruit. These are more slowly absorbed.

To obtain a net digestible carbohydrate number, take the total amount of processed carbohydrates and subtract fiber and sugar alcohols. Some experts recommend that you only subtract 50 percent of the sugar alcohols from the carbohydrates. Also, some health experts don't worry about small numbers of either carbohydrates or fiber (three grams or less), but when I am calculating, I just subtract them all. If I have eaten three food items, one with a net of two grams, one with three grams, and one with five grams, I have consumed a total of ten grams of net digestible carbohydrates. When I am adding up what I have consumed, I do not count natural, dense carbohydrates such as those found in vegetables.

To make these calculations, you have to be able to read food labels. Not reading food labels is like jumping into a swimming pool and not knowing how to swim. It's potentially life threatening!

Timing is everything. As stated earlier, *when* you eat processed carbohydrates and when you exercise is the key to controlling your blood-glucose levels. You want to consume processed carbohydrates during the time of the day that your metabolism is at its highest. Your exercise should be timed to help burn sugar and calories during times of maximum refined-carbohydrate consumption.

The Quick Reference Guide

Omega-3 fatty acids, in addition to vitamin C, help reduce the cortisol released by our bodies. Cortisol is a stress hormone that can cause us to gain weight. The adrenal glands release it along with adrenaline.

I developed this quick reference guide to help fellow patients stay organized and focused in their assault on diabetes, excess weight, blood pressure, and cholesterol, and to help them manage their triglyceride levels.

The Problem: **Excess Weight**

The possible causes—Consuming too many processed carbohydrates and too much sugar, cell inflammation, lack of exercise, excess calorie intake, excess fat intake, leptin resistance (a weight-regulating hormone), an excess of cortisol in the body (due to stress), and possible food allergies.

The possible responses—Do LRIT (low-resistance interval training), have capsaicin with dinner, chlorophyll (eat green), and seven hours of sleep daily; watch your diet—eat good fats, good carbohydrates, lean protein, fiber, and acidic foods; and avoid or limit soy, wheat and gluten, and fast foods.

Count calories and limit daily intake of processed carbohydrates and sugars to thirty grams per day, consumed between noon and 8:00 p.m. Only eat after 8:00 p.m. if you haven't exceeded your daily calorie intake. Take five hundred milligrams of vitamin C each morning and evening, and take omega-3 fatty acids in fish-oil pills or eat small amounts of olive and canola oils, black olives, walnuts, almonds, flaxseed meal, and cold-water fish, such as tuna.

Don't forget: Zero-calorie and negative-calorie foods are foods that have no significant calorie content. They are often referred to as "free" foods. Yellow mustard would be an example. Negative-calorie foods are foods that require the body to burn more calories to digest them than are contained in the food itself. Raw mushrooms would be an example.

The Problem: **Appetite Attacks**

The possible causes—Leptin resistance, sugar or carbohydrate addiction, inactivity, and the insulin yo-yo.

The possible responses—Do LRIT ("Lower it"), reduce the amount of bad carbohydrates and refined sugars you consume, engage in safe snacking, and eat protein and good fats. In addition, keep mentally and physically active.

Note: I do not consider appetite and hunger the same thing. Appetite is a craving, while hunger is the empty condition of your stomach.

Remember: Like what you eat, not eat what you like. It takes three weeks to develop a habit.

The Problem: **Higher-Than-Normal Glucose/A1C**

The possible causes—Excess intake of bad carbohydrates and sugar, lack of exercise, cell inflammation (which interferes with insulin working effectively), and the insulin yo-yo.

The possible responses—Add fiber and acidics to your daily intake, do LRIT ("Lower it"), do safe (planned) snacking midmorning and midafternoon, and eat lots of green vegetables (think about chlorophyll; eat green). These responses reduce cell inflammation and build muscle, which burns sugar. Limit daily intake of processed carbohydrates and sugar to thirty grams per day and take vitamin D.

Remember: White foods are potentially bad. Milk, processed sugar, white processed flour and bread, white processed rice, and potatoes are a few examples. You can get the nutrients that potatoes contain from much more "diabetic friendly" foods.

The Problem: **Higher-Than-Normal LDL (Low-Density Lipoproteins, the "Bad" Cholesterol) and Triglycerides**

The possible causes—Lack of exercise and excess intake of omega-6 fatty acids or saturated fats.

The possible responses—Increase fiber intake, take full daily recommended dosage of fish-oil pills, do LRIT ("Lower it"), consume capsaicin, especially at dinner, and avoid saturated fats.

The Problem: **Low HDL (High-Density Lipoproteins, the "Good" Cholesterol)**

The possible causes—Lack of exercise and low intake of omega-3 fatty acids.

The possible responses—Do LRIT ("Lower it") and consume fish-oil pills or small amounts of olive and canola oils, black olives, walnuts, almonds, flaxseed, and cold-water fish, such as tuna.

The Problem: **High Blood Pressure**

The possible causes—Lack of exercise, excess sodium intake, and stress.

The possible responses—Reduce sodium intake, do LRIT ("Lower it"), get seven hours of sleep each night, and reduce caffeine intake.

The Problem: **Joint and Tissue Pain**

The possible causes—Food allergies, excess sugar absorption, and lack of exercise.

The possible responses—Do LRIT ("Lower it"), reduce sugar intake, and eat fiber and acidics.

Remember: LRIT ("Lower it") and capsaicin will keep your metabolism going virtually twenty-four hours per day! Capsaicin delays the release of insulin by thirty minutes. Insulin creates an appetite surge; insulin might make you gain weight. Read your food labels! Metabolism is the conversion of food into living material and into energy.

Voodoo

Health-care professionals have asked me if I had bariatric weight-loss surgery since I'd lost so much weight and stopped taking diabetes medications two years ago. The answer is *no*! Prescription drugs have their place. Sometimes surgeries are necessary. But I lost weight and beat diabetes using a nonsurgical, nonprescription-drug intervention. It will help you defeat prediabetes, type 2 diabetes, and obesity.

I have attended meetings where guest speakers have presented their programs to "help" people with diabetes. At the end, the audience is told to get their checkbooks out. One of these programs was going to cost $90 per week! The methods they used were secretive and frightening. You don't need voodoo to get healthier. I've saved over $2,000 per year in medical expenses, and my grocery bill is still about the same. I eat much more healthfully, and I'm no longer sick day after day. I am entirely free of any medications.

I have saved a lot of money by reducing my dining out. It's easy to overlook the cost of restaurant and fast-food dining, but the cost can be shocking if you add it up (both in terms of your money and your health).

The Four Bs

Slowing or blocking the absorption of sugar into your bloodstream can be accomplished by using the four Bs.

Ban It

If you don't eat a high-carbohydrate or sugar item to start with, there's no way that sugar will get into your system.

Burn It

A simple way to eliminate blood sugar (glucose) is to burn it up doing exercise. I'm not talking about grinding yourself into the ground with exhausting workouts. You can burn sugar with simple, low-resistance exercise and by simply moving around more.

Block It

This technique has been used for weight loss, but guess what? It works to block, slow down, or even stop the absorption of sugar into your bloodstream, using the fourth B which is the

Back Door

You use the one-two punch (FAA) fiber and acidics. First is fiber. Fiber slows and even blocks sugar absorption. The second is acidics, which refers to acidic foods such as plain vinegars and citrus juices (lime, lemon, and grapefruit juices—orange juice is not a good idea because of the sugar content); they *neutralize* sugar! Stick to plain, unseasoned vinegars and vinaigrettes. The seasoned ones generally have added carbohydrates and may be higher in calories.

The Three Ps
"P = (P/P)"

How do you determine if a food product is refined or processed? Remember the three Ps: if it's *Packaged*, it's *Probably Processed*. That means it's suspect.

You have to read the label to see what is contained in the foods you eat. Reading food labels is one of the most important things you can do. I think it's every bit as important as exercise.

Have you ever had someone give you something to taste and he or she said, "Go ahead and try it … It's *good* for you"?

Never taste something that is mysteriously vague. If you can't see an ingredient label for the food product, don't eat it! Would you swallow mysterious unmarked pills? Of course you wouldn't.

Learn to understand what you're eating. It will empower you to control your health destiny.

Stocking Your Food Arsenal

Learn to like what you eat instead of eating what you like. I read a story several years ago about a man who went overseas for several years. At first, he did not like the food in the country where he was living. He then realized that the local diet was very healthful, and he got used to eating it. He learned to like what he ate. When he returned to the United States, he was appalled at the poor quality of food here and continued to eat the foods that he had eaten when he was overseas.

Instead of eating what we like, we need to learn to like what we eat. It takes three weeks to develop a habit; start changing your eating habits now. Once you develop a taste for certain healthful foods, you will learn to enjoy them. Later, when you taste some of the unhealthy foods you were previously eating, you will find that they no longer taste good to you. Your taste buds can be reprogrammed within a short amount of time to adapt to new, more healthful foods.

Processed foods and sugars are designed for fast preparation and quick eating. In order for the foods to be able to be prepared quickly, a key ingredient is basically removed. That ingredient is dietary fiber. Dietary fiber is one of your safeguards to slowing dramatically the absorption of sugars into your bloodstream. Remove the fiber, and one of your body's safety nets is removed.

There are many great-tasting foods that have a very low amount of digestible carbohydrates and sugars. Some foods are actually free of tangible carbohydrates and sugars. When it comes to both losing weight and stabilizing your blood sugars, these are the kind of foods you want to be eating. In addition, you'll want to engage in light to moderate exercise.

Here's how I trimmed calories from my diet:

Calories Saved

Spray oils

Cheese sprinkles

Low-calorie high-fiber bread

Reduced coatings and breading

Take a 1,000- to 1,200-milligram fish-oil pill each evening. It also raises your HDL substantially.

One medium (60-calorie) egg in the morning increases metabolic burn.

Replace some of your salad dressings with plain vinegars and citrus juices. It's okay to add a packet of no- or low-calorie sweetener (made with sucralose) on your salad if you want it sweeter.

Light biking/walking

Eliminate corn and potatoes.

Chicken or beef broth in the evening helps in weight reduction. (Cut the portion size in half to reduce the sodium level. This product is also available in low-sodium.)

Drinking 25 ounces of green tea per day will aid in weight reduction.

Many people can easily reduce their daily calorie intake by 1,000 calories without feeling deprived!

This list is only a small portion of what's available out there.

I take vitamins B1, B12, and biotin. They increase metabolism, and this combination doesn't upset your stomach like the vitamin B complex; add vitamin D3, which helps reduce glucose levels.

You may want to eat peeled apples. Half the sugar and carbohydrates are in the peel. However, the apple peel is rich in phytochemicals. You can research this concept and decide whether or not to peel your apple.

Sugar-free chocolate and caramel toppings

Sugar-free gelatin and puddings

Sugar-free bread-and-butter pickles

Sugar-free coffee flavorings

Fresh cooked vegetables (sometimes frozen are also okay)

No-calorie sweetener (made with sucralose, not aspartame)

Liquid butter spray (xanthan and guar gums)

Light mayonnaise (either canola or olive oil)

Sea salt

Red-pepper hot sauces

Precooked egg patties (or freshly cooked eggs)

Green relish, no sugar added

Negative-calorie foods such as lettuce, onions, mushrooms, etc. (Negative-calorie foods take more calories to process than they contain.)

Low-Glycemic-Load Foods

Turkey and fish products

Sugar-free jams

Lightly salted rice cakes

Fudge pops (no sugar added)

Fruit bars (no sugar added)

Almond unsweetened vanilla drink (your milk substitute)

Tuna and other cold-water fish

Reduced-sugar ketchup

Low-carbohydrate pasta (only five grams of carbohydrates instead of forty-two)

Fresh fruits

Pearl barley

Brown rice

Walnuts, almonds, sunflower kernels

Black olives

Long-cooking oats

*Turmeric

*Curry

*Cinnamon

*Mint

*Ginger

These spices increase metabolism.

Rewiring Your Brain:
Flip the Switch That Kills
Appetite and Glucose Spikes

It's time to get "the monkey off your back." Excess intake of refined carbohydrates and sugars will create a carbohydrate addiction. After a few days, once you get over your sugar withdrawal, you will feel better, and eventually you will start looking at food without any craving or emotion. You will look at food as an energy source and will think ahead about eating nutritious foods, rather than eating foods without thinking about whether they will help you or hurt you.

When you can stand in a bakery for ten minutes and stare at the cakes, pies, and doughnuts with no emotion or cravings, then you've gotten the monkey off your back!

Another trick to try is to create "fake memories." For example, tell yourself, "If I eat that, I'll get sick" or "I ate that before and hated it."

My doctor looked at me once and said, "It's like your brain has been rewired." That was a great comment, and in a way, he was right. I beat the chemical addiction of refined carbohydrates and sugars.

Food Allergies:
Wheat, Gluten, and Soy

Is there a connection between diabetes and celiac disease? Do many diabetics tend to have celiac disease or food allergies? The percentage of type 2 diabetics with celiac is about the same as the general population, which is about 1 percent. There seems to be no evidence that prediabetic and type 2–diabetic people have a higher incidence of celiac disease. However, the percentage of type 1 diabetics with celiac disease is between 7 and 8 percent. There may be a correlation of some sort between their types of diabetes and celiac disease, an autoimmune disease. Just because you don't have celiac disease doesn't mean you don't have food allergies, though.

A leading expert recently stated that there are twenty million Americans with varying degrees of gluten intolerance. Gluten (from the Latin *gluten*, meaning "glue") is a protein composite found in foods processed from wheat and related grain species, including barley and rye. It gives elasticity to dough, helping it to rise and to keep its shape, and often giving the final product a chewy texture. Yet many people have trouble digesting foods with gluten. One patient on a television program stated that she had lost about thirty-five pounds after going on a gluten-free diet.

A word of caution to diabetics: *processed* gluten-free products tend to be high in processed carbohydrates and calories and/or low in fiber. Consuming too many processed gluten-free products can lead to elevated glucose levels *and* weight gain.

Before you decide that you are experiencing nerve damage to your stomach or intestines, talk to your doctor.

Many of your diabetes "symptoms," such as itchy skin, upset stomach, or colon problems, may be the result of allergies to foods and various chemicals such as laundry detergents and fabric softeners. It's often easy to assume that physical conditions that you are experiencing are a result of diabetes. Remember that they might not be, and don't make assumptions! Talk to your doctor.

Low-Resistance Interval Training: LRIT ("Lower It")

Exercise increases oxygen and endorphins, which make you euphoric. *This is big!* Studies suggest that moderate exercise may dramatically reduce the degeneration of beta cells in the pancreas. This helps to preserve the integrity of the pancreas.

The Amplifier Effect

Diet and exercise individually won't entirely do the job to defeat diabetes and obesity. When the two are combined, though, the results are multiplied or amplified.

You can break your exercise routine into segments. Fidgeting and pacing during the course of a day can keep your metabolism going nonstop. Simple movements, even just standing, keeps your metabolism at a higher rate than sitting, and that helps reduce your insulin resistance. The minute you sit down, your metabolic rate slows way down, to one calorie burned per minute. And the endorphins released by exercise feel great. I can wake up in a ho-hum mood, but after I'm done exercising, I feel like I can take on the world.

Note: Always consult your physician before starting any exercise program.

Interval Training

In a nutshell, this allows you to get the same exercise benefits with between 30 percent and 50 percent less time and distance. You start out at a slow pace (this works for any exercise—walking, biking, etc.). About a quarter of the way into your exercise set, you ramp up your pace for about one minute and then bring it back down to a slow pace (long recovery). About halfway through the routine, you take the workout to a moderate level for about ten minutes, then back to a slow pace. About three-fourths of the way through the set, you ramp it up again for about one minute and then bring it back to a slow pace and a long recovery and finish the workout.

Interval training maximizes the effects of the workout. I'm a fan of low-resistance workouts. Patients don't have to injure themselves pushing things too hard. Daily exercise, combined with control of absorbed sugar, guarantees stunning results against prediabetes and type 2 diabetes.

Combined with the MAID (Mediterranean anti-inflammation diet) program, low-resistance exercise should dramatically reduce your glucose levels as you drop excess weight.

Pushing the Envelope

I go beyond the suggested amount of exercise (150 minutes per week), I go under the recommended calorie intake (2,800 for men, 2,000 for women, as per the Harvard Medical School family health guide), and I don't lump all carbohydrates together. I have found that it's the *type* of exercise I do and the *type* of carbohydrates I eat that create the magic.

Activity—I like to use the term *activity*. About half of my activity is actually exercise. The other half is centered on reading. I believe in studying the enemy—diabetes—and learning how to combat and defeat it. Reading food labels and understanding what they mean is critical to your survival against diabetes. Not reading and understanding food labels is like jumping into the middle of an Olympic-size swimming pool at night with the fence locked and with no lifeguard on duty—when you *can't* swim! There's a high risk of injury or death.

Exercise—Exercise euphoria is the "double E." The way I exercise is incredibly simple. I use a stationary indoor exercise bike as the weapon of my choice. The stationary bike is simple because it is

- all-weather (I can exercise anytime, regardless of outside weather conditions);

- 24/7 (I can exercise any hour of the day, seven days a week on my own schedule);

- low impact (I have managed to avoid joint, ligament, and muscle injuries);

- user-friendly (The indoor exercise bike is relatively simple to use); and

- forgiving (There is no risk of outdoor hazards, and slight mistakes on the bike are not a great risk to my health).

A morbidly obese person can crawl onto an indoor exercise bike and do a small amount of low-resistance exercise—with a doctor's permission, of course.

I also recommend walking. Walking is one of the most effective exercises you can do. You can combine it with other exercises, and there is no cost. You can fidget and pace, keep moving, walk to your car, and walk up and down stairs.

The day is approaching that medical-insurance companies will start reimbursing, at least to a degree, the cost of gym memberships. It's about time. Patients need to be encouraged to exercise. It's a long-term journey. It takes years to get to where you want to be with your health. You need all the encouragement and support you can get.

A Stronger Pancreas

Beta-Cell Preservation

Following my suggestions can have a therapeutic and/or protective effect on the pancreas. I believe I've done just that with LRIT and an exercise bike over the past three years!

Your beta cells in your pancreas are the insulin producers. The less insulin that your body requires to handle the processing of glucose (blood sugar), the less work for your pancreas. My pancreas "cruise control" should be on for the rest of my life. Over the years, the beta cells degenerate and die. They can never be replaced. What if we could slow down or virtually stop the degeneration of the beta cells?

What could possibly accomplish this? Studies are suggesting that *moderate exercise* is the key! Interestingly, the best results are obtained from moderate-intensity exercise. These findings suggest that exercise has a therapeutic and/or protective effect in diabetics. It decreases oxidative stress and preserves pancreatic beta-cell integrity—that is, it slows down the degeneration of the beta cells.

I'm maintaining an A1C under prediabetic levels constantly, with little effort. Guess what? I've been doing moderate exercise (biking) for years.

Has it paid off or what?

Five Key Hormones You Should Know About

Cortisol—It is released by stress; combat it with omega-3 fatty acids, vitamin C, and low-resistance interval training (LRIT).

Ghrelin—Its release triggers appetite; counter its release with fiber, lean protein, and good-fat consumption.

Leptin—This hormone is released from the fat cells to signal the brain that energy has been sent to the cells; the brain may be "leptin-resistant" and may not recognize the signals; using exercise (LRIT) gets the brain to start receiving the "all's full" signal.

Insulin—Insulin should only be released in small amounts when needed; it should not be wasted. It triggers appetite and weight gain. Capsaicin delays the release of insulin by thirty minutes, essentially flipping off the appetite (not hunger) switch by controlling the release of ghrelin, insulin, and cortisol and improving the brain's reception of leptin signals.

Insulin is produced by beta cells in the pancreas. Beta cells can degenerate and become depleted over time. Studies indicate that moderate exercise has the potential to increase beta-cell numbers. You could make your pancreas healthier. *What a thought!*

Glucagon—This hormone has the opposite effect of insulin; it raises glucose levels.

Glucagon is produced by the alpha cells in the pancreas. Studies indicate that when beta cells are severely depleted, alpha cells can take over their function! Also, other stress hormones that are released early in the morning to get our system going for the day can interfere with insulin effectiveness (see resources).

Timing Is Everything

To combat diabetes, it is essential to understand that much of a person's glucose-level fluctuations are the result of imbalanced food combinations, poor timing, and inadequate exercise.

To overcome this, you need to develop a sense of "plate balance." That means that your meals need to have balanced portions that include the "healthy" fats—those containing omega-3 fatty acids— lean protein, and natural, dense (complex) carbohydrates. Portions need to be measured and controlled. Dense, complex carbohydrates can be eaten in sizable quantities.

Daily exercise is also essential. My weapon of choice is an exercise bike. Each individual needs to find a type of exercise that he or she likes and will stay with. Day after day, week after week, month after month, and year after year, with daily exercise, anyone can become healthier.

Other tips to remember:

- Working to reduce your post-meal evening glucose levels can help to offset your early morning readings.

If your dinners contain a sensible amount of processed sugars and carbohydrates, and your bedtime snacks consist of lean proteins and good fats, and you maintain moderate body mobility, you should see surprisingly good glucose readings each morning.

- Grazing is good. Your metabolism has to work at burning up the food you're eating; therefore, your metabolism stays elevated.

- It's not *how much* you eat but *what* you eat that counts.

Add foods rich in chlorophyll to your daily diet—*in addition* to your normal food intake.

If you eat healthful, "diabetic-friendly" foods, you can eat *more* food, not *less*!

Don't try to starve yourself. That's a recipe (no pun intended) for disaster!

Do Your Best

Each day our "best" is different. If you feel great, you will get lots done. If you're sick, you won't get much done. Don't beat yourself up. Do the best you can on a bad day. There will be plenty of good days.

Don't make assumptions about your health. Get answers from your doctor and diabetes counselors. If you don't have a doctor, find one!

Don't take your prediabetes or type 2 diabetes or excess weight personally. There are millions of us fighting the same battle. I will be looking over my shoulder the rest of my life, watching out for diabetes or obesity to attack me again. I'm confident, but I will never let my guard down. This is a small price to pay to be healthy and virtually off all my medications.

Remember, if you believe that you'll only get sicker, you indeed will.

Get serious about fighting your condition, and don't give up!

Questions and Answers

Q: Can I eat after 8:00 p.m.?

A: Yes, if you haven't exceeded your calorie intake for the day. Avoid processed carbohydrates and sugars after 8:00 p.m.

Q: Will resistance training help me lower my glucose levels?

A: *Yes.* Prediabetes and type 2–diabetes patients who use resistance training often see reduced glucose levels. Combined with low-resistance interval training, resistance training is a powerful weapon against diabetes.

It is recommended that you have a fifteen-gram serving of protein within forty-five minutes of finishing your morning exercise routine. This will enable your muscle cells to repair themselves, and it should help you in weight loss.

Q: How many calories should I consume each day?

A: Ask your doctor. Set targets and goals with your doctor. You can go online and review the calorie guides put out by the United States government.

People tend to underestimate the amount of calories we take in and overestimate the amount of exercise we do. But be careful not to set your calorie intake too low! Your body will save the calories for "protection."

Q: Should I avoid fast food?

A: Yes, avoid fast food at all times! It has high levels of saturated fat and sodium, which are bad for your blood pressure. It is usually high in starches and sugars. If you do eat at a fast-food establishment, be aware of what you're eating. Ask questions of the staff. If you're not certain of what the ingredients are, don't eat the food item.

Q: What are the benefits, if any, of capsaicin?

A: This compound is found in cayenne and jalapeno peppers. Generally, you will see cayenne pepper in the capsules you take (usually 12,000 micrograms or 120,000 thermal units). Jalapeno and cayenne peppers are varieties of chili peppers, and all chili peppers contain capsaicin. Capsaicin has health benefits for diabetes. It delays the release of insulin by about thirty minutes. Hot, spicy foods tend to rev up our metabolism. Check with your doctor *before* you consume capsaicin!

Q: Does metabolism or the burning of calories really change much whether I'm sitting down or casually moving?

A: Once you sit down, your metabolism immediately slows down to just a single calorie burned per minute.

Wonderland

Imagine a place where you can eat everyday foods that you find at the grocery store and those foods enable you to improve your glucose readings, blood pressure, weight, good and bad cholesterol, and triglyceride levels, plus alleviate joint and muscle pain to the point that your doctor starts reducing your medications. You may stop taking some or even all of your prescription medications. You feel better than you have in years, and the good part of it is that you know exactly how you are accomplishing this feat! You've turned the clock back, and you're healthier than you have been in years. You can't believe the changes that you've gone through. Things just keep getting better.

Welcome to wonderland.

The "diabetes-reversal techniques" described in this book will help you change your life for the better. My doctor still considers me a type 2 diabetic with the disease under control with diet and exercise. I don't feel like a diabetic anymore. I like to refer to myself as a "type 2 R." The R is for "reversed." I feel healthier than I have been in thirty years. I may never need diabetes medication again! I'm *well*, and that's what matters. *Don't* get hung up on definitions and terminologies.

Health Warriors

Making a healthy lifestyle "change" is too much for many people. It's often overwhelming and uncomfortable. Your new healthy lifestyle has to be slowly broken in like a pair of new shoes. Eventually, it will be as comfortable as that favorite, well-used, comfy pair of shoes that you never want to throw away.

I'm an advocate of slowly changing your lifestyle. Trying to lose weight rapidly and keeping it off is much more difficult than slowly taking it off and keeping it off. When you have many problem areas to deal with, such as prediabetes or type 2 diabetes, excess weight, high blood pressure, and poor cholesterol and triglyceride levels, you may find that correcting them all at once over a short period of time seems next to impossible. You must patiently work at fixing the problems, bit by bit. You will be surprised by how quickly you will see results, but remember, it probably took you years to get into the condition you're in, and it will take a while to get yourself healthy again.

I refer to individuals who have taken the first step to make themselves healthy again through a healthy lifestyle transition as "health warriors." I salute them for their determination.

Good Hunting

It's time for you to quit allowing yourself to be victimized by prediabetes or type 2 diabetes. It's time to become aggressive in fighting an enemy that, by now, you know how to defeat.

You now know how to limit the intake of processed carbohydrates and sugars. You know how to ban and burn up glucose (blood sugar). You understand the benefits of the Mediterranean anti-inflammation diet and using light-resistance exercise combined with low-resistance interval training. You no longer have to live in fear of diabetes. You also know how to slow and to block the absorption of sugars into your bloodstream using the "back door," which is fiber and acidics.

Fiber is found in vegetables (and fruits, to a limited degree); acidics include plain vinegars (not processed vinaigrettes, which have extra carbohydrates) and citrus juices, such as lemon, lime, and grapefruit juices.

You also know that acidic foods neutralize sugars. You now know how to rev up your metabolism and how to prevent glucose spikes and high levels of glucose in the early morning (dawn phenomenon). You know that chlorophyll can clean up your tissue and muscle cells, which, combined with exercise, can greatly reduce if not stop insulin resistance. You won't need much insulin to do the job of balancing your glucose levels.

You've been told it's not good to live in denial. Sticking your head in the sand and denying that you have medical issues such as prediabetes, type 2 diabetes, high blood pressure, excess weight, high bad cholesterol, low good cholesterol, and a high triglyceride level is dangerous. These factors combine to put you at a significantly elevated health risk.

Arming yourself with knowledge, setting up a game plan with your doctor and your certified diabetes educators, and deciding to fight diabetes and beat it is *not* living in denial.

I've heard that diabetics can go on a medication "holiday" for a while but that we will eventually get worse and be back on diabetes medications again. I've been off all of my diabetes medications for two years. *I don't subscribe to the belief that you can't effectively and permanently reverse diabetes.*

I can't go back to my previous lifestyle—I don't want to go back to it—and neither will you, once you get a taste of "freedom" from the terrorist control of diabetes.

Summary

As you have probably noticed, my food list is full of items that are low in processed carbohydrates and sugars and are gluten-free. If you use my system correctly, it's almost impossible to fail. Between slowing and blocking the carbohydrates being absorbed by your bloodstream and burning and neutralizing sugars and cranking the metabolism, you deliver a deadly one-two punch to both obesity and diabetes. An increased intake of chlorophyll (eating green) helps to greatly reduce insulin resistance by reducing cell inflammation and swelling. Add low-resistance interval training, and you should start feeling better immediately.

You should be totally armed to take on and defeat your prediabetes, type 2 diabetes, or obesity problems. In this book, you've read about the possible causes of your condition and the possible solutions to reverse those conditions. You are now in charge. In fact, you always were. Now you have the will, the means, and the knowledge to stare diabetes in the face and say, "I can see you. I know what you are. I'm not afraid of you. I'm taking you down!"

It's payback time! This cowardly disease attacks soft targets. It hits and runs. No one is safe against it. There is no mercy for men, women, children, or the elderly. This terrorist will kill you if it can. It's your choice: either you go down or it does.

No longer will you be the victim. You will take charge, and, with the help of your doctor and diabetes educators, you will develop a plan for grinding your prediabetes or type 2 diabetes right into the pavement.

Your confidence level will dramatically increase. Instead of feeling sad and hopeless, you will have a sense of well-being and happiness, having achieved one of the greatest victories in your life! No longer will you fear lab tests and going to your medical exams.

You've chosen a healthy lifestyle for the rest of your life. Congratulations!

You will become the hunter and diabetes the prey. I wish you good hunting.

Conclusion

I've gone through a long journey in my fight against diabetes. I'm one of the lucky ones; I came out alive and well from the greatest battle in my life. Watching friends and family die from the effects of diabetes was almost too much for me to endure. I had to do something about getting the word out to all of the other patients that there's hope— that there's a way to turn your health around and live a full, happy life. Remember, if you don't have good health, you've got nothing. Financial wealth means nothing if you're medically bankrupt!

I would like to invite you to join me in helping others after you have made yourself well. There are millions of people out there who need our help. If you can help a few people fight diabetes, and they help a few more, and so on, together we can create a wave of individuals to fight this terrible disease. Get involved in your local diabetes support groups, workshops, and training programs. Many of them are free, and the only thing you will invest is time. I've invested about three years and over a thousand hours of time reading, studying, and researching diabetes topics. I've spent thousands of hours exercising. I wouldn't trade what I've done for anything.

Yes I'm at total war with diabetes—and I won't rest until it's eradicated for good.

About the Author

In 1998, my weight had hit a high of about 350 pounds. I was wearing size 52-waist pants, but my true waistline was about fifty-six inches. The shirt I was wearing was a size 3X. I could no longer keep the 2X shirts buttoned. I kept one of my 2X shirts that I occasionally wear when I am talking to diabetes patients; I also have a pair of 48-waist pants that for a time I could not wear. They are scary to put on, believe me.

From about 1992 to 1999, I had to use a BiPAP machine set at 16(I)-9(E), due to hypoxia. Fortunately, I did not have sleep apnea. The doctor said that because I was getting some exercise, my tested oxygen level at sleep was still 97.5 percent. I finally lost enough weight to be able to get off of the machine, after about six and a half years.

Just over eleven years ago, I was diagnosed with type 2 diabetes. I spent ten years battling raging A1Cs and ever-worsening blood-glucose readings. About two and a half years ago, I started developing the beginning stages of retinal problems and was sent to an eye specialist. I had lost about a hundred pounds, but I was still morbidly obese.

The reason I came to the diabetes-education arena is to help educate patients who are fighting obesity, morbid obesity, prediabetes, and type 2 diabetes with diabetes reversal.

I brought my weight down to safer levels (175 pounds), and I have been off all diabetes medications for two years. Currently, my waistline is at about thirty-four inches. My fasting glucose is just under 100, and my A1C is 5.6—under prediabetic level.

My system has been relatively simple but incredibly effective. I developed this system to help other patients. It is nonsurgical and involves no prescription drugs. This system utilizes a Mediterranean-style anti-inflammation diet combined with low-resistance interval exercise. It targets control of specific carbohydrates within a certain period of time. By eating everyday foods that you find at any grocery store, you can combat your insulin resistance. This is not a low-carbohydrate, low–fat, or high-protein diet. It's a well-balanced diet rich in natural, dense carbohydrates, good fats, and lean protein. The system gets key hormones to balance properly. You will eat better than you probably ever have—and you will lose weight and will probably have to have your prescription medication reduced or eliminated.

My medical file can verify my history of health decline and later diabetes reversal.

Diabetes is a terrorist; you don't negotiate with a terrorist! You have to understand the deadly threat that your medical conditions pose, but you also need to know that you can defeat diabetes.

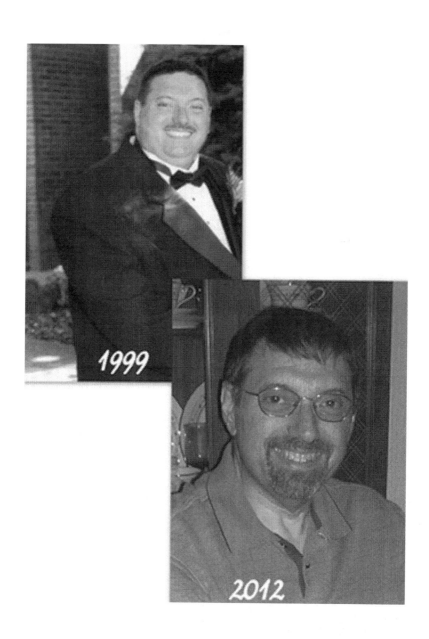

1999

2012

Resources

"Melt Off Fat," Melissa Gotthardt,
First For Women, July 18, 2011
Pages 28 through 35
www.FirstforWomen.com

"How Doctors Lose Weight," L. Maxbauer
First For Women, August 29, 2011
Pages 36 through 41
www.FirstforWomen.com

"Body Weight Set-point
Discovery," Melissa Gotthardt
First For Women, October 10, 2011
Pages 32 through 37
www.FirstforWomen.com

"The Day-Off Secret That Melts Stubborn Belly Fat," Melissa Gotthardt
First For Women, October 31, 2011
Pages 32 through 37
www.FirstforWomen.com

"Nutrient Combos that Melt Super Stubborn Fat," Michael Solan and Melissa Gotthardt
First For Women, December 12, 2011
Pages 28 through 33
www.FirstForWomen.com

"Soup Melts Away 10X More Weight," Melissa Gotthardt
First For Women, January 23, 2012
Pages 32 through 35
www.FirstForWomen.com

"Discover Your Mind/Body secret," Melissa Gotthardt
First For Women, February 13, 2012
Pages 32 through 37
www.FirstForWomen.com

"The Burning Question," Kate Lowenstein
Health Magazine, November 2011
Page 24
www.health.com

"You Can Beat the Big D," Gina Shaw
Health Magazine, November 2011
Page 95
www.health.com

"Make Over Your Metabolism", Paige Greenfield
Health Magazine, January/February 2012
Pages 45 through 50
www.health.com

"The Other Diabetes," Elizabeth Hiser
Copyright 1999

"Living Well with Diabetes," Krames Patient Education
Copyright 2011
www.krames.com

American Diabetes Association
www.diabeteseducator.org

American Association of Diabetes Educators, A.A.D.E.
(Local Diabetes Educator Referral System)
www.diabeteseducator.org/diabeteseducation/definitions.html

"Does Vinegar Control Type 2 Diabetes?—a List of Acidic Foods to Help Lower Blood Sugar Levels," Beverleigh H. Piepers
www.ezlnearticles.com

"Effects of Exercise Training Intensity on Pancreatic B-Cell Function," *Diabetes Care*,
American Diabetes Association
Vol. 32, Number 10, October 2009
www.diabeteseducator.org

"Foods that Reduce Blood Glucose"
Livestrong.com
www.livestrong.com

"Get the Most Out of Your Workout in the Shortest Possible Time!"
Interval Training
CHOICES Health Education & Wellness Program
August–September 2008
Vol. 1, Issue 2
www.choiceshewprogram@doh.state.fl.us

"Glycemic Load Index," David Mendosa
www.mendosa@mendosa.com

Nutrition Graphics
www.ngcatalog.com

"Good Nutrition: Should Guidelines Differ for Men and Women?"
The Harvard Medical School

www.health.harvard.edu

Joslin Blog, Joslin Communications
September 23, 2011
www.joslin.org

Pull-Out Reference Guide

THE MAID (Mediterranean Anti-inflammation Diet) with LRIT (Low-Resistance Interval Training) Healthy Lifestyle Transition Program

QUICK REFERENCE

THE PROBLEM	THE POSSIBLE CAUSE	THE POSSIBLE RESPONSE
Excess Weight	Consuming too many processed carbs and sugar; cell inflammation; lack of exercise; excess calorie intake; excess fat intake; leptin Resistance; body releases cortisol due to stress; possible food allergies	LRIT (Lower it); capsaicin with dinner; chlorophyll (eat green); 7 hrs sleep; eat good fats, good carbs, lean protein, fiber, and acidic foods limit/avoid soy, wheat, and gluten; avoid fast foods! Count calories; limit daily intake of processed carbs and sugars to 30 grams per day (consume them between noon and 8 p.m.). You can eat after 8 p.m. if you haven't exceeded your daily calorie intake. Take 500 mg vitamin C each morning and evening.

Appetite Attacks	Leptin resistance; sugar; carb addition; inactivity; the insulin yo-yo	LRIT (Lower it); reduce bad carbs and sugar; safe snacking; eat protein and good fats; keep mentally and physically active.
Higher-Than-Normal Glucose/A1C	Excess intake of bad carbs and sugar; lack of exercise; cell inflammation (which interferes with insulin working effectively); the insulin yo-yo	Add fiber and acidic foods to daily intake; LRIT (Lower it) Safe (planned) snacking (midmorning and midafternoon) Eat lots of green vegetables (chlorophyll—eat green). This reduces cell inflammation. Build muscle (muscle burns sugar); limit daily intake of processed carbs and sugars to 30 grams per day; take vitamin D.
Higher-Than-Normal LDL and Triglycerides	Lack of exercise; excess intake of omega-6 fatty acids/saturated fats	Increase fiber intake; take full daily recommended dosage of fish-oil pills. LRIT (Lower it); consume capsaicin, especially at dinner; avoid saturated fats.
Low HDL	Lack of exercise; low intake of omega-3 fatty acids	LRIT (Lower it); consume fish-oil pills and small amount of olive and canola oils; consume black olives, walnuts, almonds, flaxseed, and cold-water fish (such as tuna).
High Blood Pressure	Lack of exercise; excess sodium intake; stress	Reduce sodium intake; LRIT (Lower it); 7 hrs sleep/night; reduce caffeine intake.
Joint and Tissue Pain	Food allergies; excess sugar absorption; lack of exercise	LRIT (Lower it); reduce sugar intake; eat fiber and acidics.

NOTE: LRIT (Lower it) and capsaicin will keep your metabolism going virtually twenty-four hours per day! Capsaicin delays the release of insulin by thirty minutes. Insulin creates an appetite surge; also insulin may make you gain weight. Read your food labels! Metabolism is the conversion of food into living material and energy.

THE 3 P'S

THE 4 B'S

IF IT'S PACKAGED, IT'S PROBABLY PROCESSED

BAN IT, BURN IT, BLOCK IT using the BACK DOOR: fiber and acidic foods.

Lettuce with vinegar and citrus helps block the absorption of sugar—eat your salad **BEFORE** your main meal..

21574577R00067

Made in the USA
Lexington, KY
18 March 2013